WEIGHT LOSS - SIMPLIFIED

EVIDENCE-BASED ADVICE
CREATE YOUR OWN PLAN

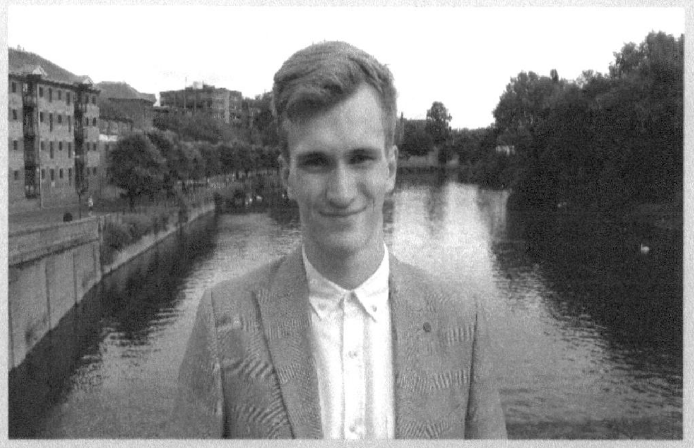

Author: Joe Harmon

CONTENTS

WHY 'FAD DIETS' DO NOT WORK

Before answering the question of the title, lets explain what a 'fad diet' means…

A fad diet is a specific diet that does not last for a long period of time, often between 1-6 months. These types of diets often have set rules for you to abide by, for example you cannot eat dairy, grains, processed foods, etc. Simply eliminating food groups that for most, are foods you enjoy and struggle to go too long without, making this specific diet approach, unsuitable for you. The process of these diet is, you lose weight initially and begin to trust the diet then often lose the weight too quick. Failing to learn any actual healthy habits to sustain weight loss, get stuck at a certain weight, do not know where to go, then your weight often slowly reverses back up.

I have tried a lot of these 'fad diets' before I became educated and started educating others. The one thing I learnt over time was all these diets normally have one or two decent principles. Most of these diets promote portion control, increasing awareness of foods and calories, so they can supply a benefit. However, if you stick with one for too long, you will often get stuck and progress will be halted, often leading to reversing back into old bad habits with foods... indulging in the foods you have eliminated for 6 months like a teenager with their first glimpse of independence!

The biggest problem these diets have is they have no education system in place to improve people's knowledge, often not justifying their approach, just a load of brainwashing and good marketing. There are no coaches or good, well-educated coaches that can support, provide empathy and educate people so they know better, maybe even be able to be independent with their own diets and lives. Personally, if I have a client more than 6 months, I feel I have failed. My role is to EDUCATE people to be able to be flexible and independent. To explain simple nutrition principles, JUSTIFYING my every decision with EVIDENCE, again to further their knowledge! Send journals and articles to read in spare time. To help create a plan to reach a goal, that is specific to their lifestyle, their food preferences and which I feel will benefit them for the remainder of their life, not just the current month!

Fad diets often consist of brilliant sales teams and amazing marketing, using your most loved celebrities to trick you into believing they have the magic answer, consistently having you pay them money because you believe this rubbish. By not educating you, by not justifying their approach or their product, you consistently have to keep paying them, for as long as you believe it is working, when it is not! Until you become educated, you will not know right from wrong!

Some diets out there, tell you to eliminate dairy from your diet. What if your mid-afternoon snack is a Greek yoghurt with fruit and you thoroughly enjoy this snack. It gives you no digestive problems or health issues. Your new diet approach says you cannot have it, now you have to have carrot sticks and guacamole instead, which you don't like. You are now eating a snack you don't like, causing you to be unhappy, therefore, you will struggle to adhere to this approach for a long time. Potentially indulging in other foods, you do like as well as the carrot and guacamole snack, increasing the likelihood of you losing your calorie deficit required to lose weight.

A similar method these diets use, is to eliminate processed foods from your diet, when I think this I think of the vegan/vegetarian diets. The principles are great, do not get me wrong, the idea of eating 100% whole foods, providing far more nutrient dense foods is great. However, this approach is not for everyone. Telling someone that only one way will work, will do so much more harm than good. Telling someone they cannot have chocolate, crisps or cakes anymore quite often will work for a week or maybe even a month, then they will give up and all of a sudden, the secret stash of chocolate is re-opened. You need to be open-minded, educated and realistic! It would probably be more realistic for you to have a certain allowance of chocolate per week, while still maintaining a calorie deficit, with a focus on nutrient dense foods, making up the majority of your diet, rather than saying chuck all your processed food away.

Some of the myths which are somehow still being floated around are no carbs/calories after dark or 6pm. If you have eaten your required calories by that time then fine... but if you have saved 600 calories for the night, because you know you are hungry and likely to snack at this time, you

WILL NOT gain fat by eating them at this time! It may affect your morning weigh-in, if you do this (read Tracking Your Progress) because the food may not be digested or excreted and holding onto water weight... but NOT FAT! Often if you eat closer to bed, it can help you sleep better... I personally have porridge before bed and I sleep like a baby.

Apparently, carbs and fats, are still bad for you. I cannot believe, this is still been thrown around some conversations I overhear, even more worrying from coaches! Let me make this simple for you, carbohydrates are your body's preferred energy source and often people who have low carb diets are very moody, unhappy and stressed. You will lose concentration, you will have decreased energy in your training sessions and will be very tired! Fats are the most calorific macronutrient at 9kcal/g, which is why so many fad diets promote low fat, because it's the easiest way to decrease calories significantly, meaning initial weight loss is achieved, you believe this is your solution and then all of a sudden you want a chocolate bar, a peanut butter sandwich, an avocado but you have been told 'fat is bad' so you feel you cannot have it. Leading to restriction of foods you can have and like before, will lead to indulgence in these restricted foods at some point. The pure misinformation being shared is causing you to be so confused and give in to these idiots, just after your money!

Have you ever seen an advert claiming, 'you must eat this to lose weight' or 'take this pill and lose 7lbs in 7 days'? If you hear this or similar phrases, you know it's a fad diet promotion! Let me tell you now, there is only one thing you NEED to lose weight... it is called a CALORIE DEFECIT! You do not need a specific food, supplement, shake to lose weight. You do not need to eliminate any food groups, unless you have a diagnosed intolerance! There are so many tips and approaches you can take which may work for you, which I will explain in later chapters.

Everybody has an approach that will work for them, often it is the most flexible approach. The majority of people who should have a strict calorie intake or meal plan are sporting athletes, aspiring sporting athletes, bodybuilders and the minority who do actually enjoy eating 100% clean foods. The majority of people cannot live this way, they may have barriers like money/finances, food availability, time, social life etc. The way you eat needs to be enjoyable, suitable for your goals, sustainable for the long-term, causing as little stress as possible and if possible, with as little food focus as possible in the future.

Stop being brainwashed and looking for the simple way! If you want to be healthy and live happily in the LONG-TERM future, do yourself a favour and read, become educated, track your foods and drink, learn a bit more about calories and how they impact your weight, if you are not losing weight, reduce your intake or move more, but do not worry ill explain this in much greater detail later on.

This book is not going to give you a quick fix, I apologise in advance if you thought it would do this and you may as well stop reading now if you think I am about to give you a way to lose a stone in a week… I don't do that crap here! The only quick fix I can offer you, is that you quickly learn that calories in vs calories out is the simple equation for weight loss and weight management, however there is more to that, to obtain your optimal health and I am going to explain everything for you!

Over the course of this book you will become educated on how to lose weight, maintain your ideal weight and be as happy as possible in the process. I will explain components of your diet that may or could be changed to optimise results and the same for your lifestyle and physical activity.

But please know this...

What works for your mates, celebrities, PT's, probably will not work for you... simply put, their lifestyle is very different, they may have more spare time, better access to foods, less commitments etc that makes it somewhat easier for them... DO NOT focus on them, DO NOT compare yourself to them... FOCUS ON YOU!

By the end of this book, I promise you will be more educated on the truth about nutrition, you will have a basic understanding of nutrition principles, which will then allow you to create your own starting plan to build from, using the steps provided. This book will show you how you can be flexible with your nutritional approach, what is actually important and how to make your life easier and your journey more enjoyable. I will show you how to manage your weight, still have a social life, eat convenience foods when necessary, have less stress and more happiness, while still eating towards your desired goals.

This is the start of your new lifestyle!

CALORIES DO MATTER

As mentioned in the previous chapter, the ONLY thing that matters in terms of weight loss, is that you burn more than you consume... a calorie deficit. Being healthy, is a different topic completely, you can technically eat McDonalds every day and lose weight, however this does not make you healthy!

You have 4 macronutrients, which provide the greatest amounts of energy/calories. These are carbohydrates, fats, protein and alcohol.

Carbohydrates

Carbohydrates contain 4 calories per gram consumed. As a whole, carbohydrates are the most dominant nutrient consumed (Jebb, 2015), due to most processed foods and preferred foods being carbohydrate dense, which explains how the original myth of 'carbs are bad' or 'carbs make you fat' arrived, to help people moderate or control their carbohydrate intake or choose better sources. However, the quantity of carbohydrates alone, does not independently cause weight gain (van Dam and Seidell, 2007 and Yunshenga et al, 2005). When the proportion of carbohydrates were increased, without increasing total calorie intake, there was no change in weight (Sartorious et al, 2017). Actually, the same study reported greater energy, satiety and mood in higher carbohydrate intakes. Although the amount of carbohydrates does not directly affect weight gain, the choice of carbohydrates could potentially play a role (van Dam et al, 2007). By eating highly palatable foods, you will then struggle to eat nutrient dense foods, due to these foods being quite bland in taste. It is not a lie to say that caramel rice cakes taste a lot better than carrot sticks, however having balanced taste buds to be able to eat both can have a positive effect on weight management. When choosing carbohydrate-based foods, try to make the majority of them high fiber, greater volume and less palatable, therefore not relying on really tasty foods, that are a lot easier to overconsume. I am sure you would agree, it is easier to overconsume caramel rice cakes than it is to overconsume potatoes.

I am sure that since this study by Malik (2006), people are more aware that there are calories in drinks like Coca Cola, Fanta and alcohol but I am sure some people still are not ware that all drinks except water, contain calories that accumulate towards their total energy intakes. When tracking your foods, please be aware that the drinks you consume besides water, contain calories that if not tracked, can be a reason why you are gaining weight unexpectedly through your eyes. All I can say is be more aware of food labels, they are there to help you!

Fats

Fat is the richest source of energy of the four macronutrients, containing 9 calories per gram. It is evident that consuming a lower fat diet significantly increases the chances of weight loss, simply due to the number of calories consumed in comparison. It is also a lot easier to overconsume calories by having a higher fat diet, due to the low satiety rating of higher fat foods.

A systematic review of 33 studies (Hooper et al, 2012), examining the effect of reducing total dietary fat intakes on weight management, showed that by simply reducing the dietary fat, showed a small but significant reduction in total bodyweight and body fat percentages. This study was based on subjects that had a baseline fat intake of 28-48% of their total daily intakes. Although, proportion of macronutrients when calories remain the same, does not affect weight loss alone, it is fair to assume that if your diet consists of nearly half your dietary intake from dietary fat, that your overconsuming calories, if your goal is weight loss.

Lower fat diets typically are higher carbohydrate diets. However, due to being less than half the calories, it is a fair and ideal replacement. However, it is key to remember that fats are vital in our diets. Ideally, when low in trans fats, intakes up to 40% of intake can be healthy, but on average 20-30% is a healthy average.

Protein

Protein, like carbohydrates has 4 calories per gram. A lot of people know and are aware that protein is responsible for growth and repair of muscle tissue, yet there are so many reasons why protein is important in our diets, even more so in weight/fat loss diets.

Firstly, protein has a higher Thermic Effect of Feeding (TEF) at 20-30%. This means that for every 100 calories you consume through protein, 20-30% is burned through the heat your body creates to digest these foods. Compare this to the 5-10% carbohydrates burn and 0-3% fat burns, you effectively burn more calories in a higher protein diet (Leidy et al, 2015).

Having a higher protein diet has many potential benefits including better energy metabolism, meaning your ability to utilise energy is more efficient. It helps regulate your appetite, as protein takes the longest to digest, out of the 4 macronutrients, helping you to feel fuller for longer, thus overall reducing your calorie intake, supporting your goals of achieving a calorie deficit.

To further this, higher protein diets also prevent a decrease in resting energy expenditure (REE), therefore you are able to eat more food in the long run (Halton et al, 2004 and Eisenstein et al, 2002). This is through muscle retention. As muscle burns calories alone, you will simply need more calories to maintain your current muscle mass, which should be music to your ears.

After consuming high protein meals, satiety hormones were elevated, blood pressure and waist circumference was decreased and reduced triglycerides were reported as well (Leidy et al, 2015). Long-term weight loss, fat loss and muscle retention were reported in participants who followed a protein rich, calorie restricted diet, compared to a low protein calorie restricted diet (Leidy et al, 2015).

You can lose weight on a lower protein calorie restricted diet; however, you will do so, on a lower calorie diet, making it a lot harder to adhere to in the long run. The results of the study by Leidy et al (2015) showed that your ability to adhere to a protein rich diet is key, for long-term results. Those who gradually increased protein over time, experienced the greatest long-term results (8+ years). Both Leidy et al (2015) and Wu (2016) reported that the ideal protein intake should be based on activity levels. Suggesting that 0.8g/kg bodyweight is enough for sedentary individuals, 1g/kg bodyweight for minimally active individuals, 1.3g/kg bodyweight for moderately active individuals and 1.6g/kg bodyweight for very active individuals. Another approach which is more realistic, is to have protein intakes at between 30-40% of total calorie intake. Although this is more generic, the previous equation for overweight/obese individuals, will massively overestimate protein requirements. Another option, if you can work out your lean mass (using body fat scales), times your lean mass by 2.2-3.1g/kg lean mass. Again, if you rarely consume protein now, increase slowly to reduce digestive issues potentially caused due to drastic alterations within your diet.

However, despite these recommendations, both studies suggested a gradual increase in protein intake over time, to help your body adjust to the higher protein intake, making it less harsh and a shock to your digestive system. Meaning if you currently consume 1g/kg bodyweight, yet you are a very active individual, training 6x per week, then gradually increase from 1g/kg to 1.2g/kg over a month, then increase again.

In older individuals who consume a lower protein diet, there is a greater risk of sarcopenia (Wu, 2016). This is the natural process of muscle loss through aging, increasing the risk of injuries, falls and decreased ability to recover. However, if protein is increased to either recommendations above or 25-30g per meal, then this helps delay the onset of sarcopenia, slows its progression and reduces its consequences. This is something to bear in mind going into later adulthood, as the sooner you consume a protein rich diet, based on your activity levels, the greater chances of delaying sarcopenia.

There are suggestions that evenly distributing protein intake across your meals and a snack, promotes the greatest levels of satiety and has shown the greatest results in weight loss, maintained over longer periods of time (Leidy et al, 2015 and Wu, 2016). Aiming for 25-30g per meal is a good starting point for most people. Typically, breakfast is a low protein meal, lunch is slightly higher, but not greatly and tea is the highest protein meal of the day. Therefore, there is a lot of potential room for more protein in our diets. It will be a case of finding foods richer in protein that you enjoy eating.

Alcohol

Alcohol has 7 calories per gram. I am going to start off by saying that you can lose weight while still including alcohol in your diet... you do not have to exclude alcohol completely. Chances are if you drink every other night and binge drink on the weekends, then yes, you will have to cut down on the alcohol. However, again all you have to achieve is a calorie deficit!

Most bottled lagers are less than 150 calories, which is less than most chocolate bars in terms of calories. I am in no way, saying that alcohol is healthy, I need to make that

VERY clear. I am simply stating that for some people, a new lifestyle choice with 1-2 drinks of alcohol per week will be a lot more sustainable over years to come, than cutting it out completely. I would say that if you can eliminate alcohol from your diet and it does not negatively affect your social life or your happiness then please do so, I am just saying again, it may not be the right option for everyone.

If you are a heavy drinker and over 400-500 calories come from alcohol per day or every other day, then a change is most definitely required for health reasons. Just having 300-500 calories per week from alcohol is a lot healthier, meaning you have more calories from solid foods, helping you feel full and in control of your appetite.

Nutrient Timing

For the majority of people who train once per day, with a general weight/fat loss goal, nutrient timing is not important. Meaning it does not really matter when you consume your calories, as long as you achieve a calorie deficit overall. Therefore, do not stress if after your training session, you have not eaten a meal within the first hour... that's ok! You are not training for another 24 hours, so you have plenty of time to refuel your body to train again the next day.

Nutrient timing is only important really for people who train more than once a day, sporting athletes who require the greatest amount of energy for a specific 2-3 hours of a day and those with serious fat loss goals, including the likes of bodybuilders. Having said this, it is known to be beneficial on satiety readings to have meals evenly distributed, however as I mentioned at the beginning, this may not work for you, based on your lifestyle and commitments. Eating 2-3 times per day may be more beneficial and adherable long-term for you. It will take time to find out your ideal plan, but you will have a good starting point to make minor adjustments to, by the end of this book.

Tracking Your Calories

I am a firm believer that even if it is for only a week or month, everyone will benefit from tracking their calorie intake. It has so many benefits that out-weigh the one negative people claim to always use... 'I don't have time'.

Even if you only tracked your intake for a week, you will be a lot more aware of how many calories you are eating, how many calories are in foods you eat every day, plus whether or not you need to adjust your calories to reach your goal.

So many times, there are people who claim to eat healthily, they eat all the foods and drinks that come under the umbrella term 'healthy' yet wonder why weight is not being lost.

It is quite possible to eat 'healthy' foods and still gain weight. You can very easily overconsume nuts, avocado, olive/coconut oil, seeds, peanut butter and hummus which are all classified as 'healthy' yet are extremely calorie dense food options. Hence why tracking your intake can be so beneficial and eye opening if you eat a lot of these foods daily.

You can eat 'healthy' foods, because they are healthy and not enjoy them, which very often leads to either overconsuming this 'healthy' food to try and find satisfaction and help you feel good about yourself or you eat this unsatisfying food and eat something really sweet, probably calorific to get rid of the taste. Think back to the yoghurt/fruit and carrot sticks/guacamole swap in the first chapter. You need to find a balance of foods that provide satisfaction to your taste buds, nutrient quality and food volume to optimise your diet.

I strongly suggest that if you are very new to this and have never tracked a calorie in your life, to make time to track your calories for a week, learn more about what is in your foods, even if it is just the calories. It will be extremely beneficial. In the long run, if you track for a decent length of time, you will become very aware of the calories in foods, making tracking your foods, less of a priority because you KNOW and have a greater KNOWLEDGE and ABILITY to make BETTER DECISIONS!

Use an app like MyFitnessPal which has the option to scan the barcode of your foods, making it even easier and less time consuming than it is already. I promise you, after the first few days, once you are used to tracking your foods, it takes less than 5-10 minutes of your day... everyone has that amount of time spare.

But please remember, drinks have calories too! Track them as well!

HYDRATION

Everyone knows that water is important, we all know that we should be drinking a lot of fluids to stay hydrated, yet so many people fail to stay hydrated. This down to numerous reasons including, people think that only water counts, even though diluted fruit juices (no added sugar) drinks still count towards this, as well as milk, a couple of tea and coffee's also count towards this accumulated fluid total. The only fluids that do not count are alcoholic drinks and caffeinated drinks in excess of 200mg per day (equivalent to 1 monster energy or 2 coffee's). Linked to this, people also do not like water, I am in that boat, but just because we do not like water, doesn't mean we have to be dehydrated, drink weak squash so you have some taste, that's what I do. I personally drink 1L everyday pure water and then around 3-4L diluted squash.

Water is no doubt up there with the highest importance in nutrition, we cannot survive a couple of days without it. Your hydration will determine how optimally you function. You can eat all the right foods and lose weight; however, you will be very miserable and lethargic if you are dehydrated in the process.

Water helps to regulate our body temperature, this is why in hotter climates when abroad or on the rare occasion in the UK we should drink more to keep our temperatures from rising too high. When we train, we produce a lot of heat as well which, again we need water/fluids to help keep our temperature at a healthy baseline level.

To help with feeling lethargic/tired, fluids help transport nutrients around the body to our working muscles, helping us to function both mentally/cognitively and physically as well. Therefore, the better hydrated you are, the more efficient your body is at digesting and utilising the nutrients you consume properly. Removing carbon dioxide from the working muscles as well, decreasing or delaying fatigue. Plus, it helps flush out the waste products via the kidneys through urine.

For those who care about their looks, water also improves the quality, strength and look of our nails, hair and skin. Also, for people who exercise frequently, performing high impact exercises, as well as older adults, or younger adults looking to improve their joint health (basically everyone!), you should be drinking enough water to stay hydrated and support your joints. Water acts as a shock absorber for your joints, therefore improving your ability to train injury free. By having sufficient water flowing around your body, you are basically optimising your health in more aspects than you are possibly aware of, so all I can say is just drink more!

To add an example about water acting as a shock absorber, try to think of anyone you know well or even yourself. Do they have bone/joint problems or aches? If yes, do they drink a lot of fluids? If not, there is a very strong potential reason. Dehydration may not be the lone reason, they/you could have worn joints out through jobs/work or other aspects of life, but your hydration is something you can definitely control and help rule out any further or potentially initial damage to your joints.

For serious gym goers or if you just want to be stronger in the gym, then you are going to want to be hydrated! Without sufficient water, your power output decreases significantly, meaning your ability to train for long periods is reduced and for the time you can train, it is a lot less effective. You simply will not optimise your strength capabilities or progressions if you are dehydrated, especially in and around your training sessions. On average, 40% of gym goers are dehydrated during their training sessions, do not be one of them!

It is important to remember that thirst kicks in, when you are already dehydrated. Making it also very important to understand the difference between thirst and hunger, or better yet not allow yourself to become dehydrated in the first place and risk being confused. Ever heard someone say, have a glass of water before you have a snack? There is a reason for that. Quite often, when thirsty you are confused and feel hungry and unfortunately quite often people choose to eat instead of drink. By eating a chocolate bar or your chosen snack, you are at no point quenching your thirst, so eventually you will feel thirsty again, probably choosing to try and satisfy this feeling with another snack... it does not work! Of course, it is natural to choose food instead of water, but it is not going to solve your problem. The best thing you can do, is drink often throughout the day, so you do not risk this feeling and confusion.

You can monitor your hydration through your urine. If your urine is very clear, you are hydrated and should look to keep drinking consistently to maintain this level. If your urine is yellow(ish) or darker then you need to fill your water bottle up and start drinking to get in a better place with your hydration. The benefits are clear. If you want to function properly at work in terms of cognition and function properly in the gym and progress without feeling tired, if you want to decrease the risk of injuries and maintain a healthy body temperature, efficiently function the way your body is supposed to, then start thinking of ways to stay hydrated.

A few ways are to get a 2L water bottle, get a permanent marker and write 8am/10am/12am/2pm on one side then 4pm/6pm/8pm/10pm on the other. This helps remind you and gives motivation for where you are supposed to have drunk by at a certain time. That way you have consumed a minimum of 4L fluids each day. Another way you can try is to set a reminder on your phone every 15-20 mins to take a gulp of water/squash… this may not be suitable for many though. You just need to find a way that works for you, a way that will remind you that you need to drink often!

A very rough guideline for water/fluid intake is:

Males – 3.6L
Females – 2.6L

Men typically have more water in their bodies compared to women, therefore require a bit more to maintain their water body levels. This is a very rough guideline to start with. You can adjust accordingly, based on how you feel. If you feel tired and lethargic, drink more than this. If you train very intensely and frequently, sweating a lot, then drink more than this. Bu at least this gives you a starting point with a few motivational tips to help you stick to it.

MONITORING YOUR PROGRESS

There are so many different ways to track your own progress, you have progress pictures, scales, bodyfat, how your clothes fit, mood books, training log books and you can even monitor your digestion, there are so many options and the more ways you can track, the more data you have to compare and identify progress and the more accountable you can be.

For example, your body weight could have stayed the same one week, but you have decreased bodyfat, you feel happier and have progressed your training since... therefore if you were just tracking your weight alone, you could get pretty beat up, but you have actually made really good progress. Look at the list and choose which ones are the most ideal for you and least time consuming if you have a tight schedule, but I am sure everyone can do at least two.

There are ways that you can optimise your results, comparability and reliability when tracking your progress. With all of these tracking methods, the more you can keep things the same, the better you are able to compare. Therefore, progress pictures, take in the same room, same time (lighting) and the same clothes. This is because believe it or not, some mirrors are different, timing matters because you can look a bit different from morning to evening after a full day of food and clothing matters because you could wear a smaller pair of jeans one time, which make you look bigger. It is just a lot easier and less stressful on your mindset to keep things the same. If not, you may find yourself confused sometimes as to why things look different.

As for scales and bodyfat measures, I would personally say that if you cannot keep things the same for the 24 hours leading up to your weigh-in, it can be very hard to have accurate and comparable results. Let me apply some context. You weigh yourself weekly on a Saturday, but you weigh yourself at different times each week. Your baseline or starting weigh-in, you weighed first thing in the morning, in light clothing before eating/drinking, then following week you weigh-in on the evening, on a full stomach in jeans and a hoodie, yet wonder why you seem to have gained 2-3lbs, yet eaten really well and have actually maintained a calorie deficit. For this example, you are likely to have gained a combination of water weight, your stomach is full of food and fluids and you are wearing heavier clothing. Scale readings are the hardest to monitor and understand if you do not know all this.

It takes 3500 calories to lose or gain 1lb, chances are you have not eaten in excess of that much in 24 hours, so do not worry, it is not fat, or at least not all of it. If you are to optimise the readings on your scales, I would try to copy the same foods and fluid quantities in the 24 hours leading up to your weigh in, having your last meal at the same time, the night before if possible. This will give you the most comparable results, potentially least stressful as well.

Although weigh-ins are the most common and seem to be everyone's choice for progress monitoring, there are a lot of other trackable ways which are a lot easier to do and understand. Like I say, if you want to do weigh-ins, I would say track your bodyfat % and take progress pictures as well.

KNOWLEDGE & FOOD FOCUS

The Power of Knowledge

Throughout this book, I will emphasise the power that knowledge can provide. Knowledge alone will not be enough, sometimes occasions happen, sometimes life happens, however if you have a good knowledge about what is right and what will work for YOU, then you have a much better chance of making a better decision, than if you did not have a good, sound knowledge.

You do not have to be an expert, you just have to start reading, you have to start challenging peoples advice, rather than accepting it and being a yes man, you have to remain or become open-minded, you have to trial and error for a while until you find your perfect balance, you have to understand that you will never know everything, that you will always be a student. The moment you think you know everything, is the moment you stop progressing, improving and become stuck again. That goes for everything in life!

The more you know and understand, the easier your choices will become, you will know what is right, what is wrong and what an ideal middle choice could be. For example, you know that a home cooked meal with sweet potatoes, lean beef mince and a small burger bun with onions and mushrooms will be the right choice, you know that going to McDonalds with your mates and having a big mac, with large fries, a milk shake with an ice cream is the wrong choice, however, going to McDonalds with your mates and socialising and having either a happy meal, wrap with small fries, burger with no fries and a diet coke is a middle/suitable option that allows you to socialise with your mates, but not having a significantly different calorie meal that ruins your calorie target for the day. It is very possible to have a balanced social life, meanwhile still achieving your goals. You just have to be smart. To be smart you have to be educated. To be educated you have to learn. To learn you have to read, track your foods, invest in yourself and your goals!

Some people would rather stay in and have the first option, but some would rather go out with their mates… I am just showing that if you were to go out with your mates, you can still have a balance. I will keep providing examples that EVERYONE is different, everyone's lifestyle is different, stop comparing and wishing you had someone else's life, focus on making yours better!

Food Focus

Having emphasised that knowledge is a very big reason and impactor on your decision making, I now will talk about food focus, how to manage this healthily and the normal transition period as you begin learning, begin being more independent with your diet and ore flexible in time.

As you increase your knowledge, become more aware

about food and your choices, your food focus will increase. This is normal, typically the more you know about something, the more you tend to care about its impact on yourself. Ultimately, what you do not want to see happen is your food focus remains so high and intense that you start eliminating other aspects of your life, like social occasions. This is why it is vital to learn a balance, for example choosing the middle option in the example above every now and then, is perfectly fine, probably healthier for you than to stay in every night.

To start with, you will probably choose to stay in and choose the healthiest option, because you have not learnt how to find that middle ground occasionally yet, or you are trialling out your new approach, to increase the amount of whole foods in your diet, both are perfectly fine. During the early stages, this is normal and somewhat expected. In coming months however, you will want to start finding a balance between work, food, gym, family, friends and social life experiences, so that you can have what is called overall optimal health. Yes, nutrition plays a big role in your health, but it is not alone. I assure you, if you can occasionally find that middle ground of an ideal meal choice with friends and family, you will be a lot happier than eating at home 365 days a year. Even bodybuilders and sporting athletes do not live that strict. Think of it like this, as long as all of your decisions, lifestyle choices and food/drink habits have a positive average, you will certainly be heading in the right direction. Meaning it is sometimes ok to eat out, sometimes ok to have an ice cream or indulge slightly in your comfort foods, doing so probably makes your new lifestyle choices a lot easier to stick to, if you are allowed this little indulgence. This is why people who cut out food groups that they enjoy, tend to eventually over indulge in these restricted foods at a later date. Learn moderation, portion control and what you can afford to consume, that will satisfy you as well as help support you in reaching your long-term goals.

For some having a little bit of chocolate each day makes life easier, some people will have a pizza on a Saturday night. Whatever helps you stick to your plan, find a way that works for you. A small example using the Saturday night pizza option can be, you know after tracking pizza last week, that the pizza you want is 1000 calories, your calorie goal is set at 1700. You have a few approaches you can take. You can cut back foods on this day leading up to your pizza and have 700 calories across the daytime, indulging in the pizza on the night, or you can do more activity on this day, so you can have 900 calories across the day (+200 based on activity increase), helping create a deficit through activity rather than food alone, or you can choose a thinner pizza base, saving 200-300 calories off the pizza for the daytime. You could mix it up, week to week or a combination of 2 may work. Find your own way!

Nutrition has been made out to be very strict, one-way fits all and you will fail if you don't do this or that. I am telling you now, your ideal nutrition plan that will work for you, will be flexible, sustainable, enjoyable and one you can stick to realistically for a very long time. Focus on food so much that you begin to care about your health, understand what it requires to be healthy, but not too much that you now obsess over every food choice. There is a balance, you will find yours.

Nutrition and Mood

Nutrition can have a significant effect on your mood status, simply because it is reported that those who are overweight/obese are more likely to experience depressive thoughts and experience sadness due to their current situation, in relation, often feeling less motivation and willingness to succeed, especially in regard to health-related goals (Breymeyer et al, 2016).

Those who are overweight/obese often have less self-esteem, tend not to love themselves and feel very demotivated to do exercise based on their current fitness levels. The way to best look at it is, everyone has to start somewhere and the quickest results you will get, will be if you start right now!

Weight loss not only allows you to have more optimal health, decreased risk of physical illnesses and diseases, but also decreases mental disorder risks as well. Which is even more reason to fully commit to yourself. Be selfish sometimes and choose your own goals, because you have to come first, especially when it comes to your own health.

Dietary recommendations are to reduce sugar, if consumed at the moment in excess. Reduce total fat if exceeding 40-50% of total calories and base foods on a lower glycaemic rating, including wholegrains and higher fiber foods. Along with increased protein intake as well. Finding the balance between feel good foods for your mind and feel good foods for your body is key, for finding the overall balance for your health.

HEALTHIER EATING HABIT TIPS

<u>Shopping</u>

Meal Plan and Make a List: By meal planning what meals you are going to have for the week ahead, you will be able to provide a full list of the foods/drinks you will require to make these meals. Your meal plan and shopping list will be affected by the time you have available to prepare the meals. Probably who you are cooking for e.g. whole family or just yourself. Therefore, take all of this into the equation when creating a meal plan for the week.

However, it is very hard to plan 7 days in advance for meals, due to plans changing, time available changing and many other variables that can alter your capability to stick to a plan. Therefore, to make life easier and also increase your activity in doing so, try just buying foods for the next couple of days instead of the whole week. The pros of this idea are that you will have the chance to be more active. Either walk to your local supermarket that has sufficient food sources for you or park a bit further away, if you must drive to your store. You are a lot less likely to have food waste, as you will have a better idea of your plans and time available over the next 2-3 days than the next 7. The only potential downside is if you are a huge impulse buyer, then spending more time shopping could increase your spending. However, this can be controlled, you just need to say two simple letters together… an N… and an O… NO, when you come up against something you want but do not really need! Relish the above benefits if you continually waste food each week and are stuck for ways to increase your activity, outside of the gym.

Only Use Isles You Need: This is very common shopping advice and I am sure you have all come across this at some stage of browsing the web at ways to stop buying foods you do not need or to simply save money. Yet, people still go down the chocolate, crisps and alcohol isle every time they food shop, despite their cupboards already being stocked up at home!

As I mentioned earlier, you just need to get a stronger mind-set and say NO! Continually think of your goals like it is an obsession! You must succeed, you must overcome this but to do so, you need to think… will buying this help me towards my goal or will it make me take two steps back? In this case your goal could be to save money yet spending an extra £10-15 a week on stuff you really did not need, will not help you and add that up over a year, you are spending £520-780 extra which could go towards a family holiday, a new car or to just have as savings. If you need any motivation to prevent further impulse buying, look at how much extra you spend a year… now think how much better you could have spent that amount or maybe, not have spent it.

If you do not need bread/confectionary/alcohol/freezer

products, simply avoid these isles, save your money, support your goals and when you have achieved your set goals, reward yourself with a little break, a new car or something as a reward with the money you have now saved up.

Do Not Shop Hungry: Again, this may be one you have heard of before, the whole chew some gum while you shop or drink water as you walk around. These are all good ideas, all promoting ways to steer you clear from buying unnecessary foods you may not necessarily need.

When you are hungry and you go food shopping… all of a sudden you start thinking how to solve your hunger now, rather than what you need to buy for the week. Then all of a sudden, a chocolate bar creeps into your basket, with some crisps and a load of food you want, simply because your appetite is through the roof and you want everything in sight. If anything, you are better off shopping when you cannot stand the sight of food, the last thing you want to do is eat… that way you are more likely to only purchase what you NEED, rather than £20 extra of which you want, that will not help you.

Like most things, it is trial and error for what works for you. Try chewing gum as you shop, if that does not work, try drinking water as you go, if that fails then try shopping straight after a meal, if that fails, shop at the end of the day, when your stomach is full and just want to get home and go to bed. You may also want to try shopping alone, to prevent impulse buy temptations from others. All these things can be effective, it is just finding which is most effective for you.

Cooking

Struggling to Reduce Calories: Try grilling your meats instead of pan frying them in oil. If you do not like grilled meat, then either fry with 0 calorie sprays, or use your desired oil, but use kitchen roll to wipe away excess once heated.

Instead of store-bought frozen chips, make your own. If you don't have time, then prepare the potatoes a day in advance and keep in the fridge or make in bulk and freeze until required. Do not let time be a barrier! Get ahead of the game and get prepared! Again use 0 kcal spray or oil but removing excess.

Buy low fat versions of foods. I can hear some of you saying 'but the low-fat stuff is bad for you, because artificial stuff is used'... if your goal is weight loss, you are struggling to lose weight and consume full fat milk, yoghurt, cheese and so on, then moving to low fat options is your next step. Low fat options are only bad, in some cases when you are failing to get sufficient fat in your diet. Which if you consume nuts, avocados, hummus, fattier cuts of meats, seeds etc, then you will not fall short of dietary fat, by turning to lower fat alternatives. I will cover artificial sweeteners in coming chapters to explain the confusion, plus how they should be used, if needed in your diet.

Nutrient Retention: For optimal nutrient retention, you want to minimally cook vegetables as much as possible. The more you boil most vegetables, you are better off drinking the boiled water, as all your nutrients are in there now. The best cooking method is steaming, but I am aware not all will have steamers or can modify saucepans to create a steamer. So, my advice is to boil the vegetables just enough so you can eat them, that way you have retained as much nutrients as possible. An example of a nutrient that is destroyed by heat, is vitamin C.

Meal Prep: I understand that all out 7-day meal preps are not for everyone, myself included. However, everyone can benefit from preparing certain meals on certain days where we know we are busiest. That way, we prevent getting something from the local café, a local takeaway or being peer pressured into doing so either.

Take a look at your weekly schedule, when you are working, when you have commitments and responsibilities. Now identify which of these either or both offer a time constraint, or you are likely to be tempted by an unhealthier alternative for your goal. These are the times and meals that you need to meal prep to help support your goals. For some people, that is every lunch for 6-7 days a week. For some it is different every day, but you need to identify these times of your week, so that you can prepare the meals, making your life easier when it comes to reaching your goals!

However, educating yourself on convenience foods that are healthier and offer you some value for your satiety levels will definitely help because you may forget one day to prepare your lunch. This is when you need to know what a decent alternative is. Such as a better than average meal deals or having rice cakes with hummus and cooked meat. There are loads of convenience foods, that are not at all unhealthy, that can actually support your goals. So, do not be afraid of convenience foods, just know which ones can offer you some benefits.

Food Volume: Food volume is often something people overlook and underestimate when going through their personal weight loss journey. It is important to know that, although calories in vs calories out, is the greatest determining factor for weight loss, there are so many other elements that should be understood and managed within your diet. Technically you could eat a large fish and chip takeaway every day and lose weight, as long as a deficit is retained, then gain weight eating cucumbers all day that in total, exceed your maintenance calorie requirements... however, which is going to make you feel more satiated? Of course, it is the cucumbers. Why? Think how many cucumbers you would need to eat to over consume your calories? It would take around 100 cucumbers to consume 1400 calories!

Back to reality and the point of this chapter. Use the above example as an eye opener and take a think about what it is telling you.

Although, you could lose weight eating all the calorie dense foods you love, that have very low nutritional benefits, but you probably will get to your calorie goal for the day, still be starving and then you are stuck! However, if you had that chocolate bar, or half each day, then focus on the remainder of your calories coming from greater volume-based foods, like vegetables, starchy/fibrous carbohydrates, as lean protein as you like and moderate fats, then this plan will most likely be a lot more balanced and sustainable in the long run.

Convenience

As mentioned above, convenience foods do not always have to be bad, however they do tend to offer unhealthier options, very calorie dense, minimal fiber and very little to offer you to help you feel full. If your meal deal consists of a 550-calorie sandwich, 200 kcal crisps and 150 kcal drink, that's a 900-calorie meal which can be consumed in 5-10 minutes. You will not feel full and will be after something else in less than 2 hours, to try and salvage a decent satiety level. Another problem is that for some, 900 calories is more than half of their calorie goal, which is why I again say, choose higher volume foods for your calories, especially when they are restricted already somewhat. You could have a 400-450 kcal sandwich, 50-100 kcal snack and 0 kcal drink, which nearly halves the previous example. Choose a sandwich without mayo if possible, one that has some salad on there and with a decent amount of protein (20g+). Choose a snack like fruit bags, popcorn or one of the 100 kcal crisps that are now available. Then choose either water or a diet drink which helps save some calories, yet still offers a sweet taste that you may be craving.

It is up to your food choices, whether convenience is bad or good for you. You can make it an ideal choice, but it can also be a bad choice. Try to get into a routine, where you are always prepared, but being aware of better food choices, if you do forget, will be beneficial... I will finish by saying, make sure you read the food labels!

Money Saving Tips

Shopping Late At Night: Not only is shopping at night a good idea, as you are tired and most full of food, meaning your appetite is normally at its lowest pre-bed, but shopping later at night, close to closing times, you are likely to benefit from reduced produce and meats, that you can freeze for later use, of up to 3 months. Supermarkets tend to reduce products that have a sell by date of the current date, which means you are likely to save a fair few £££ if you can buy your meat at these times. Personally, I lived by this rule as a university student... let me say, I saved a lot of money doing so! It is well worth seeing if you can benefit from this tip!

Utilise Cheaper Shops: In the UK, there are a lot of discounted food supermarkets that you can utilise, in comparison to those bigger stores. You are definitely better off trying to match the same shop you do at the bigger chain stores, at the discounted ones to at least see a price comparison. Most of the times, you are able to do a decent food/drinks shop at the discounted stores, then maybe doing a smaller shop at the bigger stores, buying products the smaller discounted stores do not have. Again, this has pros and cons, such as it means more travelling around and making the initial job longer, but it has a great chance to save you money and become more active, especially in terms of walking.

Pay Cash Instead of Card: It may seem very strange for some to pay cash instead of card nowadays. If you take a certain amount of cash, leaving your credit/debit card at home, you are preventing yourself from overspending. Budget yourself each week for food/drink. Take the cash out each week, that's your allowance to spend on food/drinks. It will take a certain number of weeks to get a rough idea for spending each week on foods/drinks, but once this average was been worked out, stick to it and do not pay card for food. It is too easy to pay by card, easier to impulse buy and therefore, overspend your normal limit. Try this out and see if it helps you stick to your budget and your food list as well. Hopefully it makes life easier. You will probably get frustrated for a few weeks, you will see some things you want, but now cannot get, due to being budgeted, but hopefully, it will provide some financial and possibly health benefits too.

Online Shopping: This is one, again is probably more suited to impulse buyers, who have tried the above, yet not managed to avoid those unnecessary purchases. Somehow, you are still managing to buy the latest gadget, CD, DVD or more food than you really need. Most big supermarkets offer home delivery for as little as £1 on certain days/times which is worth the money, if shopping online helps you stick to your budget and plan. Online shopping is also more suitable for those who use time as a barrier for eating well and sticking to their plan. You can book your shopping as you watch your TV in the evening, or whenever you sit on your ass for 30 mins. This option is perfect for you if, you are time restricted and turn to unhealthier convenience foods because you have nothing beneficial for you or your goals in your house, because you claim to not have had the time to shop yet.

Food Choices: The foods/drinks you decide to eat need to be based on all of the following, or at least a balance of most. You should take into consideration, your budget for food/drinks each week, the time you will have in the week to prepare foods/meals, your goals and how the foods you choose will affect your progress, your preferences (foods you actually enjoy eating) and sufficient food volume and micronutrients (vitamins and minerals).

You may look at this and either think, DAMN that's a lot to consider when buying my food each week, or say, I already do this. My response is yes, it is a lot to consider if you are stuck and have never really thought your shopping through, but overtime, you will find the balance that is required to see progress... everything with regards to your health, needs an element of patience. Use these considerations the next time you shop and think, do I actually like this food? Is this food worth the price? Will I be able to moderate this food to support my goals and satisfy my sweet tooth? It will be very strange to begin with, your shopping time may increase for a few weeks, but you will start making better decisions when shopping, which will then directly allow you to make progress in the kitchen and the gym as well! As for those who claim to already base their food shopping on these considerations, I ask you, are you seeing progress? If yes, then brilliant, continue doing as you are. However, if you are failing to make any progress, you are not being strict enough with the considerations or you are simply lying to yourself! Eat foods you enjoy, eat foods you can adhere to overtime, eat foods that help you feel full, eat foods that support your goals, while maintaining the all-important calorie deficit! Ultimately, your food choices, will directly impact your ability to stick to your plan, your happiness, your mood and your progress.

We expect results tomorrow, we take magic pills expecting all the hard work to be done for you, we want everything right now! Get this in your head right now... this WILL take time and if you still believe you can sustainably reach your goals with delusional quick fix pills/shakes, then please stop reading and go and buy the overpriced books that support and provide that crap! Then, return back to this book in 2-3 months when you failed to make any progress or gained more weight than you lost, using the rubbish meal replacement shakes and start taking your health seriously, invest time into your own health. Get educated and make your life EASIER!

NEAT

What Is NEAT?

NEAT stands for Non-Exercise Activity Thermogenesis. This is typically known as activity we do, that does not have a focus on calorie burn/weight loss. Activity like walking your dog, housework, gardening, walking as you shop and even fidgeting all counts as NEAT activity. It all helps you to create a calorie deficit.

Most calorie equations do not account for NEAT activity, only the amount of sessions that you perform in the gym or specific training frequencies. Therefore, your NEAT activity, will count as an added bonus, one that you should look to optimise, to maximise the number of calories you can eat, yet still lose weight.

How to Optimise NEAT Output?

If you know that currently, you are not walking much or being active outside the 60 minutes you spend in the gym, then I recommend you take a look at your lifestyle choices and habits. How much TV do you watch sitting down? How long do you spend scrolling social media pages sitting down? How many hours do you spend sitting down at work? How long basically do you spend a day, not being active? For a very large portion of the population, the answer is FAR too much time!

I now challenge you to make a small change to your life-style. Do your usual gym routine, but for 30-45 minutes of every day, where you typically watch TV, scroll social media or just sit doing nothing, go outside and walk, put some music on or even still scroll social media, but the difference is, you are MOVING! For a lot of people, cutting out all TV and all sitting down time is impossible, I am not asking that. I am asking for a small change and for you to commit 30-45 minutes sitting down time to be converted to walking or something that requires physical EFFORT!

No matter what your lifestyle is like, I guarantee you, you have spare time, that can be spent a lot more productively! Try and stay accountable for your NEAT activity by down-loading a free pedometer app on your phone or if you have a fit watch, then start wearing it! Track how many steps you average across the week. For some, a target of 3-4,000 steps a day will be challenging, but its better than the 3-400 you were doing. Then when this becomes too easy, increase to 6,000 and so on. I bet you, if you are reading this and you are in a plateau, keep all training and food the same, but increase your steps, I bet you will start to see small decreases in weight again. Plateau's often occur because your body has adapted to the calorie balance you have been in, meaning a variable has to change. You either need to decrease food or be more active. As I mentioned before, for some, the thought of less food and more hunger is not an option, but instead of giving up, reversing back to old ways and losing all the motivation you once had, walk more outside, it sounds simple, but it really is that simple.

Typically, the aim for steps each day is 10,000 steps, but for some this is daunting and would give up, hence why we have smaller goals to start with, that in the long-term,

10,000 will not be such a daunting number, because you have already built up to 7-8,000 steps. Its important to aim big, but start small, start being realistic. 10,000 steps burn's on average 500 calories (this depends on intensity and factors including age, height, weight), but it is an average. For some, this is the difference between staying still or losing weight. For some who are losing weight already, yet feel very hungry and are struggling to stay full, despite eating more protein, drinking more water and having a higher fiber intake with decent food volume, this means you can have a bit more food, still lose weight, but help you feel full... again making the plan, more sustainable in the long-term!

Understanding Neat Expenditure

It is important to know how to manipulate your calories based on your NEAT output/expenditure. Most apps and fitness watches will give you a 'calories burned' number... IGNORE that number, no current app/watch is that advanced yet to accurately track your true energy expenditure. This goes for treadmills, cross-trainers, spin bikes, you name it... its not a true reading! That is why I urge you, to not to eat back the calories the technology says, but look to increase the time spent being active, increase the resistance on CV (cardiovascular) equipment, increase the intensity of your walks for leisurely to brisk. Use calorie burn numbers on equipment as another thing to increase, but not with a reason to eat that specific number back. Track your steps, this is the most accurate measure of NEAT, for those who enjoy being accountable and seeing progress through stats, but also those who want to make the link, to what is helping to lose weight.

I would only say to ever increase your calorie intake if:

-        You are struggling to feel full, you are finding it hard to stick to the plan and are close to giving up. I would say to create an expenditure through walking, then one of two things (or both), may happen. Either the increased activity will be the distraction you needed to take your mind off food, or you increase food by 100-200 calories based on a 400-500 calorie deficit, helping you stick to your plan.

-        If you have been sticking to your plan for a long time, you have seen a lot of progress, but you are feeling very demotivated and need a break from the focus you have put towards your goals. Take what is called a 'diet break'. Be a little more flexible with your approach, maybe increasing calories to maintenance for a few days or up to a week, enjoy this deserved break, then settle back down into plan, having had that release, with a greater drive to push forward.

-        You realise you are losing weight too quickly, personally realising you may struggle to keep the weight off and adjust to the diet long-term. Then increase your calories slightly, to promote slower weight loss. This will help you to feel fuller on the foods you eat, probably meaning you are happier too.

Hopefully, if you have never come across this term (NEAT) and what it means, or what it can do for your goals, then you can begin to utilise this within your plan. As a population we are gym potatoes. We believe that the bit we do in the gym is guaranteed to be enough. For some, it is for a period of time, for some however, you overestimate the calories burned in your training sessions.

At the end of this book, there will be a step-by-step guide to create your own plan. This will be your starting point, for you to make minor adjustments to overtime, based on the results you get. The formula for some, will not be 100% accurate, but none of them are, just like fitness watches, but they give a better, more individualised starting point, based on your age, height, weight, gender, activity level.

SUPPLEMENTS

The Confusion

The definition of supplement is "a thing added to something else in order to complete or enhance it".

Yet, people take a multivitamin and forget about ever consuming a fruit or vegetable again. Take protein shakes without ever having a food source of protein, completely misunderstanding how supplements should actually be used within a diet.

First off, to identify a deficiency you can do a few things. You can become educated about the benefits of each nutrient, understand symptoms of having deficiencies in a specific nutrient. Look to increase this nutrient in your diet, through food sources that you can enjoy/tolerate consuming and see of you experience any benefits overtime. Another option and the better, more accurate option is to go and get a blood test done by your doctor. See if there are any stand out deficiencies that can be identified. This will give you the greatest understanding of what your body is lacking. The first option is very blurry in terms of proper application. There could be a combination of deficiencies, that when trying to fix one, it feels like it makes little difference to how you feel.

Optimal Health

This is taking nutrition further than just calories in vs calories out now, because you can have a chippy a day (as mentioned before) and never consume a fruit or vegetable and lose weight, but my word, you will be very unhealthy, and your body will not optimally function at all. Your health goes so much deeper, hence why I encourage you to test to see if you have any noticeable deficiencies that should be taken care of, through proper nutrition and IF necessary, a supplement.

It is very possible to get most of your micronutrients from food sources and dietary changes to your intake, however some nutrients require regular consumption, especially water-soluble vitamins B and C. These are needed daily, as excess is excreted through urine, therefore not stored for later use, unlike fat-soluble vitamins A, D, E and K. Vitamins B and C, if not consumed daily, can lead to deficiencies overtime, causing you to feel weak, lethargic and very tired, along with digestive issues such as constipation and diarrhoea. Fat-soluble vitamins are not required daily, due to being stored in your liver for later use. Therefore, consuming foods like sweet potato, regularly every day, can lead to overconsumption of vitamin A, potentially leading to impaired vision, bone pain and changes in your skin. Hence, the importance of monitoring your diet and becoming educated on basic topics, including vitamins and minerals to understand their role within the body. All you need to do, is read a trusted government webpage on this, you will soon understand, hopefully leading to practical changes to your diet as well, if needed.

It is said, that if you are unable to make dietary changes to your diet and a noticeable deficiency has been identified by your doctor, then a supplement may be help you to increase this nutrient within your blood. When choosing your supplement, it is advised to do your research or seek advice on which ones are best. Not all supplements are created equal, they have different concentrations and bio-availability's (amount of the nutrient that can be absorbed by your body), therefore, seek advice from your doctors as pharmaceutical vitamins and minerals, are well trusted.

Nutrient Enhancers and Inhibitors

There are also vitamin and mineral enhancers and inhibitors, which is well worth taking note of. Unfortunately, it is not always as simple as just consuming the vitamins and minerals, as some nutrients act as a blocker, preventing absorption. Some nutrients also increase the absorption of certain nutrients and here a few examples.

Iron has an enhancer in vitamin C, therefore consuming a small glass of orange juice with a liver and onions meal or steak will increase the absorption of the already, highly available iron from the meat. However, as plant-based iron is not as available for our bodies, it is very important to take vitamin C, along with an iron rich meal, to optimise iron absorption, minimising iron deficiencies. This is especially important for vegans/vegetarians, that typically lack iron, along with many other nutrients that are more available in an animal product rich diet. However, iron also has inhibitors in dietary fiber and caffeine. Therefore, when consuming an iron rich meal, it is best to limit the fiber content consumed within the meal, along with eliminating caffeine before and after your meal, to maximise iron absorption.

Another example is adding 3-5g fat to a meal rich in carotenoids (form of Vitamin A), as this is fat-soluble, this increases the absorption of carotenoids, which gets converted to vitamin A when digested. An example of a nutrient inhibitor is calcium and Non-haem iron (iron found in plant-based foods). Both nutrients attach to cell walls, however calcium stays in the doorway, effectively blocking the access for non-haem iron. Advice is to take these two nutrients on separate occasions/meals. If consuming as a supplement, consume at different times as well e.g. iron in the morning with a glass of orange juice and calcium after lunch or evening time.

I hope that this chapter gives you some insight into what health actually is, how complex it can be, but also how important it is to know this kind of information, if you really want to be healthy, both on the scales and in terms of optimal bodily functions. Let me tell you, it is not hard to find this information out on the internet, you may find this all very overwhelming, it can be, but you can also learn from it. Start slowly building, step by step, throughout this book, what YOUR plan will look like. What is realistic for you, but also how are you going to get educated? You have podcasts, the internet, journals, social media, educational videos, books and so much more available... cross reference it all, apply it to yourself, relish the benefits for yourself!

ARTIFICIAL SWEETENERS

Artificial sweeteners have been around for a very long time, since the last war actually. However, have only recently in the last decade been targeted for research, since artificial sweeteners have become more and more present in our diets, aiming to reduce our energy intake.

There has been a lot of confusion surrounding this topic, even so that bringing it up in a general discussion often leads to very conflicting views, based on what others are saying and what is being spread across social media. It is common among vegans/vegetarians to dismiss artificial sweeteners as it does not follow their protocols, plus amongst older adults, it seems to be dismissed due to not being natural, like 'normal' sugars are.

So, what does the research have to say?

Artificial sweeteners have never been directly associated with weight gain, meaning, by consuming artificial sweeteners does not do anything mechanically within your body to increase the storage of fat on its own, having often 0 calories, it is impossible to gain weight. We know that now, if we did not before. Only a calorie deficit or surplus can indicate weight gain or weight loss. By consuming artificial sweeteners, it is believed to promote reduced energy intakes.

However, this is conflicted with some research by Roberts (2015), who despite agreeing that artificial sweeteners do not directly cause weight gain, they can affect people's intentions and behaviours towards their diet, in a negative way. For example, some people, when consuming sweet foods, whether artificially sweetened or sweetened by sugar, often want more of that highly palatable food. It tastes nice but takes a long time to feel full, thus why it takes so much, to finally feel satiated. It is known that food/drink is associated as a reward, often going out for meals to celebrate, having 'treats' to reward accomplishments. Observational studies (analysing people's natural behaviour) also concluded that, those who consumed artificially sweetened foods (like reduced sugar chocolate, diet drinks, cakes), did not feel the same rewarding effect, sugar-sweetened foods provide. (Roberts, 2015). There is also what is called the 'licencing effect'. This is where, people consume artificially sweetened foods/drinks, therefore think it is now ok to indulge in other foods, because of choosing artificially sweetened foods/drinks earlier on (Hubberts, 2014). The ideal approach to using artificial sweeteners, is to replace sugar-sweetened beverages and sugar-sweetened foods with artificially-sweetened drinks and foods, to replace calories, rather than add them.

Intervention studies, however resulted in reduced energy intake, thus moderate weight loss (Roberts, 2015). It is commonly reported in the few studies that have been conducted properly, that artificial sweeteners CAN aid weight loss, due to their restricted calorie nature. However, the problem mainly occurs due to lack of education of how to utilise artificial sweeteners in the diet, to support a reduced energy intake (Roberts, 2015 and Hubberts, 2014). The inclusion of artificial sweeteners in your diet, will be based on individual preference, with your reaction/response to these foods, also being very individual. However, education/knowledge is always the limiting factor.

Short-term randomised controlled trials (129 studies) have shown decreased energy intake and bodyweight, which is further backed up by sustained randomised controlled trials lasting from 4 weeks - 40 months (9 studies), showing that weight loss, was maintained across a long period of time (Rogers et al, 2016). Meaning, that when used correctly, like examples shown below, you can benefit from replacing calorie dense, sugar-sweetened foods/drinks with 0 calorie, artificially sweetened foods/drinks. It depends on your current diet, whether you could benefit from including these within your diet.

Older studies, often performed on animals have often been flawed, despite some finding conflicting results, compared to human intervention trials (Rogers et al, 2016).

So, ideally how should artificial sweeteners be used in our diets?

The first thing to consider is, what your baseline/current diet looks like and includes, in terms of sugar-sweetened and artificially sweetened calories. If you are currently consuming frequent calorie dense sugar-sweetened beverages and foods, such as fizzy drinks, cakes, sweets and chocolate, then you may well benefit from the inclusion of some artificially sweetened beverages and/or foods. For example, if you consume 1-2 fizzy drinks per day, 1 slice of cake at night for pudding and a handful of sweets, you may benefit from first adjusting your fizzy drinks to 'diet' drinks, to save anything from 200-300 calories. You could also try baking your own cake, using artificial sweetener instead of sugar, to see if that suits your taste. As I have preached throughout this book, everything will be trial and error, but gradually you will build your own 'perfect' plan for you.

On the opposite side, if your diet does not currently have a lot of sugar-sweetened calories, you tend to feel full on the foods you eat, then you may not get any added benefits from consuming artificial sweeteners.

From a hydration stand point, if you are able to drink sufficient water, reaching the minimum guidelines stated earlier in the book, then adding in unsweetened diluted fruit squash or other artificially sweetened beverages will not be needed. However, if you only consume 1L of water, because you do not like the taste, then adding in diluted fruit squash or flavoured water without any added calories, may benefit you from a hydration point of view, thus satiety rating as well.

Another approach is to only consume artificially sweetened foods/drinks when you most often tend to reach for cakes/fizzy drinks, for example late night pickers or midday pinchers, may find taking a 'diet' drink or reduced sugar cake with them instead, more beneficial, based on calories alone.

In conclusion, the use of artificial sweeteners is a very individual choice, based on your current dietary intakes and goals (Roberts, 2015). A review of reviews by Mosdol et al (2018), showed the amount of expert/unflawed research available on humans is sparse, therefore, consuming artificial sweeteners in small-moderate amounts replacing current sugar-sweetened calories would be a safe alternative, but no research has been done on extended intense consumption of artificial sweeteners, so while they are safe to consume as a weight loss aid, be mindful of the amount consumed and do not over do it.

If you can understand the above information, utilising artificial sweeteners effectively to aid weight loss and not as an addition to your current sugar-sweetener calories, then you are likely to benefit, so long as a calorie deficit is reached still.

YOU ARE UNIQUE

It is a shame, that we now live in a world where we compare ourselves to everyone else, we want a certain body, or we want to look like our most loved celebrities. We live in a world of very little patience. If something cannot be achieved in a week, we seem to not bother putting in the work, that could yield unbelievable results. We compare ourselves to others, yet do not know how different our lives are.

Let me apply some context... below are two lifestyles.

We have a very lean individual, below 10% body fat, very muscular and has what a lot of people want in terms of body image. They have a six pack, large muscles, look amazing, very athletic and aesthetically pleasing. Now let's dig beyond physical aspects. This person works as a freelance PT, who lives their life in the gym, can train several times every day, can eat whenever they can in-between clients, can prepare meals. This person has also grown up in a very active family, has grown up with a healthy lifestyle, therefore has had to make minimal changes to their lifestyle, in order to be where they are today. This person is not in a relationship, has no kids and very minimal time-consuming commitments. Therefore, outside of training their clients, they can apply all the spare time, to themselves. Can freely train more than once a day, spends a large portion of their day on their feet, meaning their NEAT is very high. Based on this lifestyle example, it would be fair and honest to say, they have a better chance of having that physique. I am not saying it was easy for these people, but I am saying, they have more time to commit to themselves.

Next, we have an average body type, around 18-20% body fat. Not as muscular, not as lean, but spends a very large portion of their day, wanting the first individuals' body. Again, let's look deeper than the physical side. This person works 6 days a week, a 9-5 office job. Already, your time is limited to invest into yourself and your physical goals. This person is married, with two kids. They have commitments to take their kids to school every morning, therefore training before work is not an option. Their kids also have group activities they do a few occasions each week. Meaning less time again to give themselves. They grew up in less active families and developed less healthy habits and lifestyle habits. Are you beginning to see what is happening here? This person is going to be far less active in terms of gym time and NEAT expenditure. They have time consuming commitments that will come before their own goals. This person probably could train 3-4 times per week, providing they are motivated enough to spend their only time in the gym and being active. They will have a lot more or different stress to cope with. This person has to help raise two kids, maintain a marriage, possibly do a job they may not enjoy, take their kids to school and activities they do on top... this person may only get 1-2 hours to commit to themselves... Let me emphasise, THIS IS OK! This is a large portion of adults and our population. The first individual is not very common, but we all know someone who lives a lifestyle around a gym. We compare ourselves to them, yet I bet if they lived your lifestyle, it would be very different.

It is ALL about doing what YOU can do!

If you can only spare 1 hour a day to exercise, then that is your way forward. Your progression will be to increase the intensity of that 60-minute session to get fitter. Your goal will be to find a way to be more active outside the gym. It could be walking a little distance to work, walking to shops with your kids. Just do what you can, be honest with yourself and I tell you now, everyone can do a little more if they try and commit hard enough.

Stop wishing you had a certain body, stop comparing yourself and start comparing yourself to who you were yesterday! Are you in a better place? Are you seeing progress? Are you losing weight? Are you happy? Are you getting progressively fitter? Are you getting more and more active? Are you becoming more educated? Are you improving yourself as much as you can? If you say yes, then AMAZING! Keep going, if you say no, then look back, make changes, SMART changes, REALISTIC changes, SUSTAINABALE changes and move forward! Be PATIENT!

Your lifestyle will be very different to most people you surround yourself with and those on social media you follow. You may not have the same time available, you may not have the same environment, you may not be as happy, but you can START making small changes, that in time, will yield very big and positive results, that you will be GLAD you made this decision right now to start.

CREATING YOUR PLAN

When creating your plan, there are a lot of lifestyle questions that you need to ask yourself and you need to be honest but also flexible with your answers.

Now the first step is using the below equation to create your ideal starting calorie goals:

Basal Metabolic Rate (BMR) Formula – Mifflin-St Jeor Equation

For Men: BMR = 10 x W (kg) + 6.25 x H (cm) – 5 x A (age) + 5
For Women: BMR = 10 X W (kg) + 6.25 x H (cm) – 5 x A (age) – 161

There are numerous equations you could use, but this version has commonly shown to be within 10% of accurate readings, meaning you will have to adjust this number a lot less, compared to other versions.

Once you have worked out your BMR based on accurate measurements of your weight (first thing in the morning at the emptiest state, as well as your height and age. The next step is to times this number by your activity level listed below. These activities are simply based on sessions of exercise e.g. gym sessions, running, individual/team sport training. As mentioned before, NEAT is not included in the equation, technically counting as extra calories burned.

Activity Level:

Little/No exercise = BMR x 1.15

Light exercise (1-3 x week) = BMR x 1.25

Moderate exercise (3-5 x week) = BMR x 1.375

Heavy exercise (6-7 x week) = BMR x 1.45

If your activity is moderate exercise, your sum will look like this – BMR x 1.375.

Now you have worked out how many calories your body burns in a day or your Total Daily Energy Expenditure (TDEE). This number is your maintenance calories based on your activity and BMR. The next step is to create a deficit that is realistic to yourself.

My own personal advice is for you to think, what amount of a deficit will you feel comfortable maintaining? For some that is 500 less than maintenance, they can maintain this comfortably, but some 500 is too drastic and based on what this equation has given you, you do not want to lose 500 calories. Therefore, a smaller 250 calorie deficit is more realistic for you. Yes, results will be slower, but you will stick with this plan for longer and be easier to maintain the weight loss, once a target has been reached.

As I have mentioned in previous chapters, you can create a calorie deficit through activity as well. Therefore, if you want to eat a little more food, you can do so, if you can commit to walking 5,000 steps or however high you set your step count target. For those who want slightly quicker results, but cannot afford to decrease calories any more, then greater activity is your way forward. On the other hand, if your calorie requirement is reasonable, you know you cannot commit to too much extra activity just yet, then you may be wiling to lose a few more calories, to create your ideal deficit and rate of weight loss, you feel comfortable with maintaining.

Although stable weight loss has been deemed most effective, for example losing 0.5-1lb per week, due to it being more sustainable for most, in the long run, when you come to maintaining weight lost. It is also perfectly fine to have staggered weight loss, where you lose 1-3lbs per week, then maintain for a few weeks. This often occurs in people with very fluctuating lifestyles in terms of available time to exercise. You may have a period of 2 weeks where you can train 4-5 times per week, then a phase of 2 weeks where you can train 1-3 times per week. This is fine, that is what could work for you and your lifestyle.

As mentioned in the calories do matter chapter, although macronutrient ratios have no effect on weight alterations, they ca still have a part in promoting greater satiety. Therefore, using the guidelines for protein based on activity levels as mentioned below:

0.8-1g/kg bodyweight for minimally active individuals
1.3g/kg bodyweight for moderately active individuals
1.6g/kg bodyweight for very active individuals

You can always use the other options of either 30-40% of calorie intake, or if you have access to a body fat scale that provides your lean mass weight, multiply this by 2.2-3.1g/kg instead to get more realistic true readings, based on your current bodyweight.

If you are consuming minimal protein currently, you should aim to gradually increase your levels to your required target, which ever you decide to go with. Although, for ease and convenience, I would use %'s. If your protein intake is currently very minimal, avoid digestive stress by slowly increasing protein. For example, if you only consume protein once or twice a day, then look at having a portion of protein at each meal, then aim for each protein portion to be between 25-30g, then gradually increase this until you reach your required protein target.

A healthy starting point if you wanted to monitor your macronutrients via MyFitnessPal, would be to have the protein goal as recommended above, 20-30% coming from fat, then the remainder from carbohydrates. If you work this out, then you can input this data into MyFitnessPal, to work it out in grams for you. This is of course optional, but it can play its part as a beginner, for understanding what balance makes you feel most energised.

For example, if you wanted to track macronutrients, you weight 90kg and are moderately active, you will require 117g protein on average, which is 468 calories. You have set your calorie goal at 1650 and have chosen 30% to come from fat, which is 495 calories, which is 55g fat. So now you have 963 calories used and 687 left from carbs, which is 172g. Please remember, this ratio has no effect on weight loss, but can help you promote satiety and can always be manipulated depending on your preferences.

Where to Go Now?

Ok, so you have worked out what your calorie requirements are, creating a realistic starting point in terms of a calorie deficit. Whether you are going to have a deficit purely from decreased foods, increased activity or a mix of both.

So, what is your next step?

You now need to come up with a plan to help you feel full, while still managing to enjoy the foods you are eating. The question you need to ask, is what is going to make this plan easier?

Will buying a small block of chocolate each week as an allowance for the week help, by having a small amount each day or every other day, to help enjoy your new lifestyle more? Or will it be best to have an initial period without it all together, because you know you have not got the will power just yet to only have a small amount?

Will having a meal like a pizza or takeaway once a week, fitting within your calorie goals help you stick to the plan, knowing you have that indulgence to look forward to each week?

You also need to find what foods that are higher in volume that you enjoy eating. What vegetables and fruits do you enjoy consuming? What carbohydrate sources do you enjoy eating, which whole-wheat varieties do you enjoy (pasta, bread, etc), do you prefer white bread, pasta, rice? If so, then go ahead use them. Maybe, to increase fiber content, have 50/50 of each type.

What protein do you enjoy eating? Are you going to eat mainly meat or are you vegan/vegetarian, therefore how are you going to get sufficient protein/bioavailable calcium and iron? Are you going to incorporate an occasional protein shake to help your protein requirements, or will this waste calories and find foods easier?

What fat sources do I like, that I can consume in low-moderate amounts to support my hormonal balances, but not over consume that it ruins the calorie deficit?

These are your important questions, that the answer may change overtime, but important to bear in mind:

What is your goal?

For some it is to simply eat better and develop better eating habits, that are maintainable, experiencing weight loss, would just be part of that process. Some may have specific weight loss goals, therefore, creating a short/medium/long term goals will help make the process less daunting. For example, you want to lose 3 stone, so try developing better habits and being more educated in the first month, making small but effective adjustments, then kick on when a realistic plan is in place and developed, based on the below questions.

How many times can I train each week?

For some this is 3 times, it could be more or less. You will all have a starting point, that will look to increase if needed to progress further with your goals, if you plateau. However, remember that your gym sessions/runs are not the only hour you are able to expend energy. Remember NEAT? Walk more, do more active tasks/hobbies. Those who are most efficient in reaching their goals, have a high NEAT expenditure.

How frequently can I realistically eat?

It may benefit you more to eat 3 bigger meals than 5-6 smaller meals, depending on your appetite and hunger levels and when you feel typically most hungry and food focused e.g. this may not be at work, but could be at 9pm when you watch TV and tend to snack.

How can I look to consume enough food volume and feel satiated?

How are you going to motivate yourself to drink sufficient fluids based on the guidelines provided of 3.8L for men and 2.6L for women? Are you going to use the 2L bottle and mark the time zones? How are you going to consume enough protein? How are you going to consume enough fiber? Plus, consume high enough volume of foods, that takes enough time to consume, to help feel full, before reaching for a pudding/sweet treat?

How much time do I ACTUALLY have to commit to my goal?

Based on your lifestyle and time-consuming commitments like work, family and social commitments, how much time can you commit to being active in the gym or other sessions you enjoy? Where can you find that spare 30-45 minutes for extra activity on top of your planned sessions? What meals do I have time to prepare and which meals will I likely have to choose a healthier convenient option?

How can I become more educated on health and nutrition?

What way do I learn best (reading or listening)? How can I fit this into my lifestyle and time I have available e.g. listen to podcasts as you do your walk? What areas of nutrition and health do I want to learn about the most?

How can I look to incorporate more vitamins and minerals into my diet?

Will eating vegetable rich stews/casseroles/soups help you consume more veg? What fruits and vegetables do you enjoy eating, what vitamins and minerals do you have covered within your diet, therefore what nutrients may you lack, thus potentially require a supplement to attain sufficient amounts? Is getting a blood test done feasible?

Are my goals, SMART, REALISTIC and MAINTAINABLE?

Have you been smart in your approach, looking to take small steps, rather than run and trip over at the first hurdle? Are there small steps in place, with a greater goal at the end? Do you look at your plan and feel like YOU can do this? Do not create your own 'fad diet'!

When is best for me to eat?

When are you most hungry (upon waking/middle of day/ late at night)? FYI if it is all times, then you have 3 meals, one at each time, with one snack possibly? When do I train? If you train upon waking, you may benefit from eating breakfast, if you train in the evening, you may benefit from having your first meal later on around 11am if you do not feel hungry when waking up. This allows you to have more energy potentially throughout your session. Also know, if you do not feel like eating when waking up, you may benefit from fasting until you actually feel hungry, whenever this may be.

How can I make my plan bearable?

As mentioned above, how can you fit your indulgence in

(one big meal out, small amount each day, etc)? What little treats can you include in your diet without overconsuming, that can make your plan enjoyable... you do not have to eat a chicken salad at each meal to lose weight, if anything you are more likely to fail, with this approach. However, having a square of chocolate or biscuit with a coffee, may making eating 2 chicken salad-based meals a lot easier.

How am I going to monitor my progress?

Again, we have covered this earlier, but which way is beneficial and most relatable for you? Will taking pictures each week, along with consistent weekly weigh-ins be your most sustainable way? Will you benefit from avoiding scales and sticking to mood books and monitoring happiness and your relationship with food, along with pictures instead? This may benefit those, that realistically cannot keep a consistent 24 hours leading up to weigh-ins and get easily frustrated. Find what will keep you motivated and what will work best for you, based on what makes you most comfortable.

How long will I track my calories for?

This one is a lot simpler... as long as you need to! For some, it will be very short-term, those who will happily eat the same foods every day and just need to modify their portions, will not need to track for too long, unless they want to adjust at some point. For those who consume a very varied diet and have never done this before, it may benefit you to consume for longer periods, to get used to a consistent calorie intake and understand what calorie values loads of different foods have. Who knows you may fall in love with it, realise it does not take much time out your day, once you get into the routine of it... you will be surprised how easy it is to use a calorie/food tracker!

How can I look to decrease my food focus overtime?

For some this will happen naturally, when knowledge goes up, gradually food focus comes down as making better decisions just become natural. For some, it will be a case of keeping busy, to distract you from focusing on food all day, this typically happens when you spend a lot of time in the house or tend to overthink, so I urge you, if you do spend large portions of days in the house and alone, develop a hobby and get out more!

Should I try artificial sweeteners?

This is very individual, as mentioned in the artificial sweeteners chapter. If you currently consume a lot of calorie dense foods sweetened by sugar, or even drinks, then it may be worth trying the swap, see how you respond and see if it supports you in making progress. If you find that it triggers you to consume more calories, then it is best to avoid this, trying to cut down and create a calorie deficit through other methods.

What foods should I eat?

Again, this is even more individual. There is no food you MUST eat, there is no food you MUST avoid (other than allergies and foods you do not like eating). The most successful plans will have foods you enjoy eating and also tolerate eating. You may be able to tolerate certain vegetables and snacks which are fine to eat but provide a greater benefit in terms of helping you eat less foods over the day. You may love sandwiches, so include them, but may tolerate other less calorie dense snacks.

Having worked out your calorie goal now, that will be a deficit that suits your needs and rate of weight loss you desire and find maintainable, along with answering all the above questions based on your preferences and lifestyle you wish to now obtain, you will be in a much better position to kick on moving forward. Having learnt the basic principles of weight loss, the psychology of setting your goals and overcoming obstacles, you are already more knowledgeable than before reading this book... however, there is still so much more that you can learn to become more educated and make better decisions.

Hopefully, this book has provided all the information for you to create your initial starting plan to go forward, making any necessary adjustments along the way, but also hopefully showing you how to decrease stress through the power of knowledge and also evidence-based scientific approaches.

CONCLUSION

Throughout this book I have preached that knowledge provides greater power, which is true. The more you know the better decisions you will tend to make, more consistently, thus yielding more consistent and better long-term results.

Just simply read more, be more active than what you are right now, whether that be longer sessions, more frequent sessions, walking more, doing more physically active hobbies, control what you eat, enjoy what you eat, but long-term you need to also enjoy the process.

You have two big variables to control to lose weight, you have nutrition and exercise. Often, you will try and out train your bad diet, leading to a yo-yo effect of dieting, greater stress and an unhealthier relationship with food. However, if you can control your food, the most difficult variable is under control, making your journey so much easier for you!

You may even start to enjoy your exercise, not see it as something that NEEDS to be done but something you WANT to do instead... just think how amazing that would feel! Make it happen.

As discussed, you have a lot of other variables that can contribute, like hydration, protein, fiber, food focus, sleep, tracking your progress, all of which have important roles, but control your food, understand why you should control your food, then you will instantly see progress!

Get educated. Get inspired by yourself. Get active. MAKE PROGRESS!

FUTURE EBOOKS:

Weight Gain – Simplified

Getting the Most Out of Your Nutrition

Making A Change

Being Happy Again

Follow my Instagram @nutritionalinstructor for more information and valuable knowledge to apply to your own life and new lifestyle!

Did you enjoy this book?

Please leave a review at www.amazon.com

References:

Eisenstein, J., et al. (2002). High protein weight loss diets: Are they safe and do they work: A review of the experimental and epidemiological data, Nutrition review.

Halton, T, L., et al. (2004). The effect of a high protein diet on thermogenesis, satiety and weight loss: A critical review, Journal of American College Nutrition.

Hooper, L., et al. (2012). Effect of reducing fat intake on bodyweight: Systematic review and meta-analyses of randomised controlled trials and cohort studies, British Medical Journal.

Hubberts, D, W. (2014). "Because I am worth it", Perspective of Sociology and Psychology Review.

Jebb, S, A. (20015). Carbohydrate and obesity: From evidence to policy in the UK, Proceedings of the Nutrition Society. 74(3).

Leidy, H, J., et al. (2015). The role of protein in weight loss and maintenance, American Journal of Clinical Nutrition. 6(1).

Malik, V, S. (2006). Intake of sugar-sweetened beverages and weight gain: A systematic review, American Journal of Clinical Nutrition. 84(2).

Mosdol, A., et al. (2018). Hypothesis and evidence related to intense artificial sweeteners and effects of appetite and bodyweight changes: A scoping review of reviews, PLOS ONE.

Roberts, J, R. (2015). The paradox of artificial sweeteners in managing obesity, Current Gastroenterology Reports. 17(1).

Rogers, P, J., et al. (2016). Does low energy sweetener consumption affect energy intake and bodyweight: A systematic review including meta-analyses of evidence from human and animal studies, International Journal of Obesity.

Sartorious, K., et al. (2017). Does high carbohydrate intake lead to increased risk of obesity: A systematic review and meta-analyses, British Medical Journal.

Van Dam, R, M., Seidell, J, C. (2007). Carbohydrate intake and obesity, European Journal of Clinical Nutrition. 61(1).

Wu, G. (2016). Dietary protein intake and human health, Royal Society of Chemistry.

Yunshenga M, A., et al. (2005). Association between dietary carbohydrate and body weight, American Journal of Epidemiology. 161(4).